Healthy Eating

Introduction to Egg and Cheese Dishes

Healthy Cooking Series

Dueep J. Singh

Mendon Cottage Books

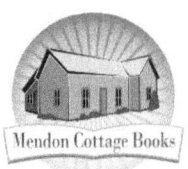

JD-Biz Publishing

Disclaimer

The information is this book is provided for informational purposes only. It is not intended to be used and medical advice or a substitute for proper medical treatment by a qualified health care provider. The information is believed to be accurate as presented based on research by the author.

The contents have not been evaluated by the U.S. Food and Drug Administration or any other Government or Health Organization and the contents in this book are not to be used to treat cure or prevent disease.

The author or publisher is not responsible for the use or safety of any diet, procedure or treatment mentioned in this book. The author or publisher is not responsible for errors or omissions that may exist.

Warning

The Book is for informational purposes only and before taking on any diet, treatment or medical procedure, it is recommended to consult with your primary health care provider.

Check out some of the other Healthy Gardening Series books at Amazon.com

Gardening Series on Amazon

Check out some of the other Health Learning Series books at Amazon.com

Health Learning Series on Amazon

Table of Contents

Introduction

One may wonder why I am writing a book on egg- cheese, because after all, this is such a common topic, and one knows all about nutritious egg and cheese combinations. But then, this book is going to tell you all about the tips and techniques with which you can eat healthy, with just some egg and cheese dishes added to your healthy diet.

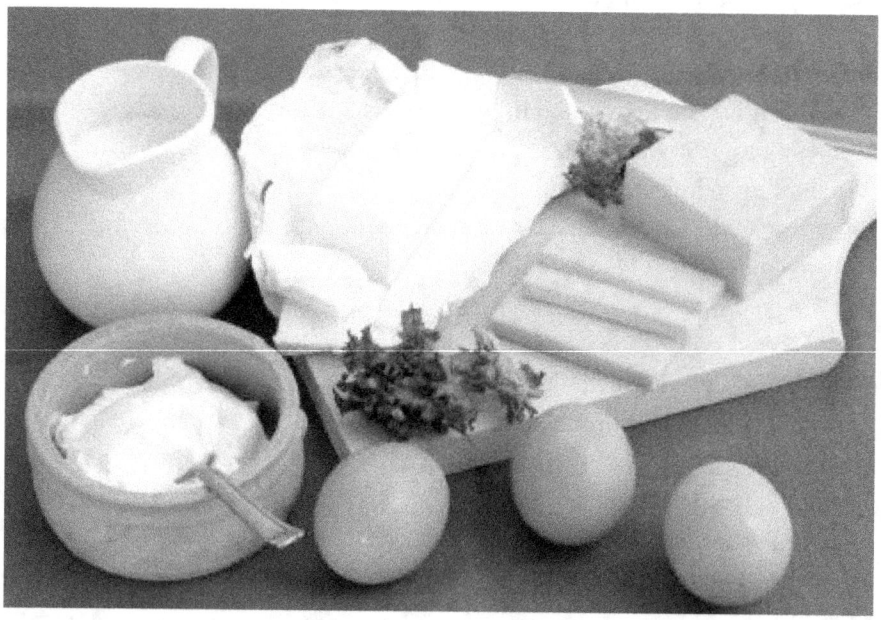

Also, a friend of mine was browsing through some of my books, and she just told me, "all these books are very interesting, but I am often based in places where I do not get these exotic herbs and spices easily. Also, sometimes my budget does not run into buying plenty of fruit and vegetables especially in these inaccessible places. At that time my larder is often restricted to just eggs and cheese."

So I started to think. Yes, what she said was sensible, and logical, because most of the time, I find myself eating egg and cheese, one because I like it, and two, because those are the items which are in the larder at the end of the month after a whole month of hectic spending and paying off the bills!

This book is for all those people, who want to know about healthy eating, especially using eggs and cheese and their combinations. These recipes are time-tested, and time-honored and have been used since ancient times all over the world, because "hen fruit" and cheese have been part and parcel of human life and the social fabric all over the world.

Eggs

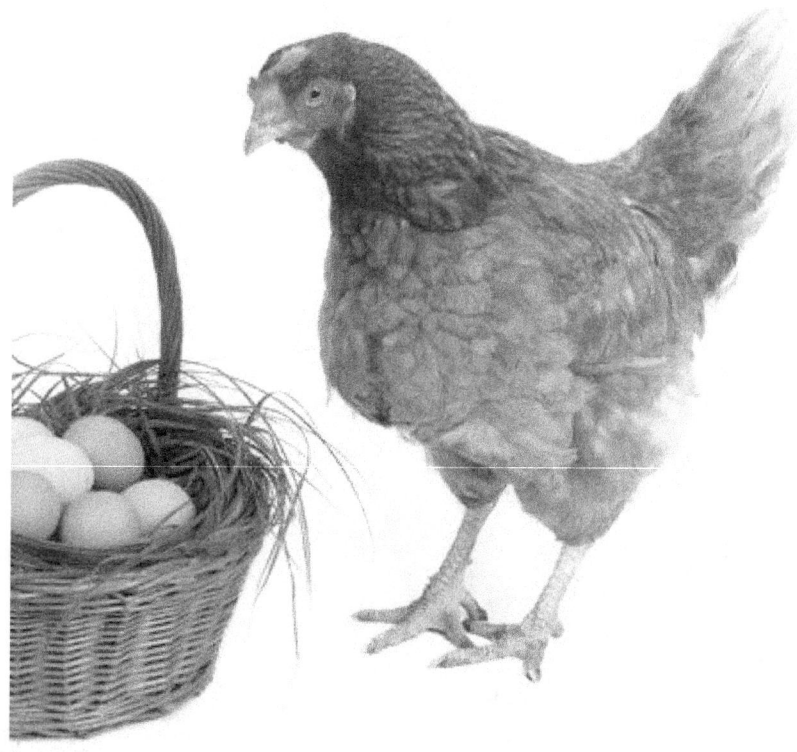

The use of eggs in cuisine globally has been lost in the shadows of time. Apart from providing nourishing dishes, eggs have also been playing an important role in general cookery as coating, binding, leavening and thickening agents. We use eggs for garnishes; we use eggs for sauces.

There are some ancient societies in the world where eating eggs are still considered taboo. For example, in some parts of Africa, the worst way to insult a woman of some particular tribe is to offer her an egg. Nevertheless, in the more civilized worlds, eggs have been in use to make delicious treats for a hungry family since prehistoric times.

It is not known when man made up a combination of flour and eggs to make egg noodles. He started using his creativity and began to make delicious omelettes and soufflés which were served as a main course. But that was when he had access to a large number of eggs. These dishes were easily and quickly made and even amateur cooks could make them with a little bit of enterprise.

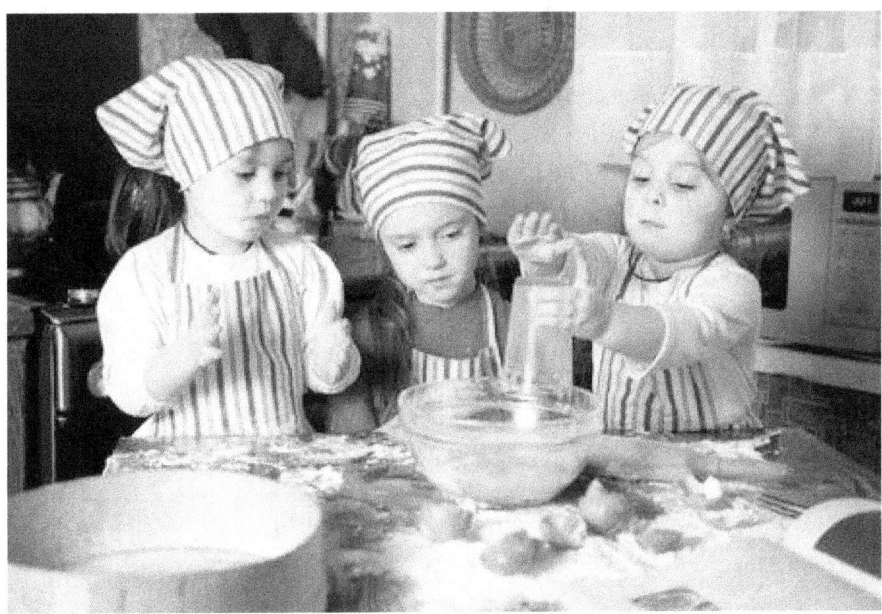

What fun!

Ancient recipes, going back to the days of ancient Rome show us how Roman cooks used eggs as a thickener for sauces, soups, stuffings, fillings for pie, and hundreds of other dishes including salad dressings. They were used as coating agents when used for dipping cutlets, croquettes and other foods for frying.

This was definitely not restricted to just Roman cookery – cooks all over the world were using these time-honored methods to make cakes, cookies and muffins, by using eggs as a binder to hold all the other ingredients together. For some types of cakes, especially those cakes which we know as sponge cakes, chiffon cakes and angel food, eggs were used as a leavener.

As a child, I was fascinated with some piece of interesting archaeological knowledge which told me that the ancient towers of Ulan Bator in Mongolia were made up of clay in which was mixed mule's milk and eggs to make solid cement. Now this was creativity of a high order!

The nutritional value of eggs has been known since ancient times. They are excellent sources of organic proteins, that is why an egg and bacon breakfast was an integral part of the start of the day for centuries in many parts of Europe.

Once upon a time, nobody bothered much about organic eggs because they knew that their eggs supply was coming directly from a farm. But as science and technology began to grow, people started experimenting with eggs, instead of leaving them alone. So now the products you get in the market are eggs, but they have been genetically improved, subjected to scientific procedures and other actions well designed to remove the natural flavor and quality of an egg.

Eggs are also used to improve the texture of frozen mixtures because they act as stabilizers and preventing lumps in sauces. For example, in mayonnaise, hollandaise sauce and other similar emulsions, eggs are used as a stabilizer.

In soups they are also used as clarifying agents.

The Chinese slice omelettes into strips to use as garnish on top of their dishes. In Asia, the garnishes normally done with sliced hard-boiled eggs.

Preserved Chinese duck eggs, known as "ancient eggs" are preserved in clay smeared earthenware pots, having been encased in a stiff coating made of strong tea and ashes and charcoal dust. Chinese omelettes are imaginatively and deliciously contrived with fillings of chicken, pork, mushrooms, shrimp and crab mixtures. The Chinese also excelled at egg reinforced noodles dishes and delicious egg custards.

So, if you're lucky enough to find best quality eggs, which are not always available in retail stores, in an organic farm, congratulations! I did not know that eggs were graded into different sizes abroad. In the East, you have just one size, – chicken egg size depending on the poultry variety!

But you are going to find extra large, large, medium, small and smaller sizes in retail stores. These are suitable for frying, soft, hard, and poaching. Some different grades are excellent for cooking and baking.

How to know whether Eggs Are Fresh

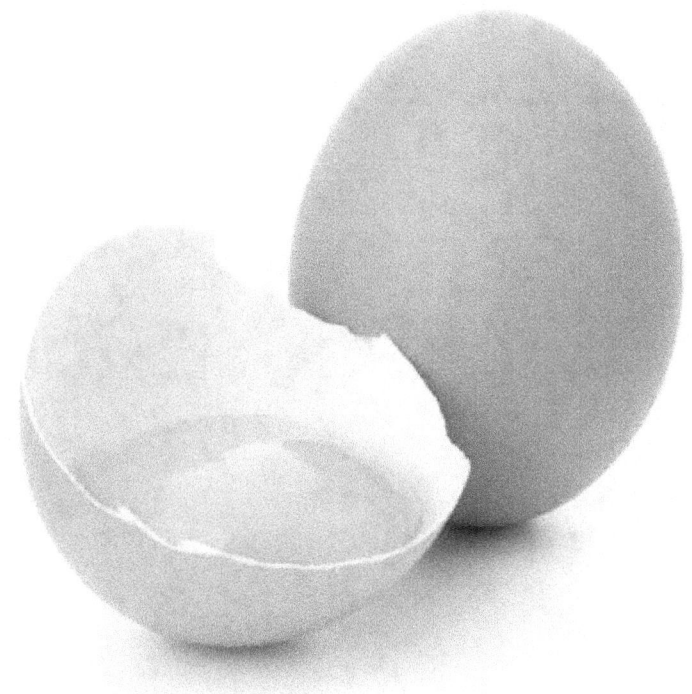

A fresh egg is going to sink straight to the bottom of a jar full of water. A comparatively stale egg is going to stand on one end, bobbing up in the water. A rotten egg is going to float on the top.

Eggs, whether they are small, medium or large can be used equally well in most cooking. In some recipes, however, actual volume of eggs are taken into consideration and you may want to look at this egg volume equivalent, which can come very handy –

You can fill an 8 ounce measuring cup with –

Whole eggs	4 large	5 medium	6 small
Egg yolks	14 large	17 medium	19 small
Egg whites	7 large	8 medium	9 small

How to Store Eggs

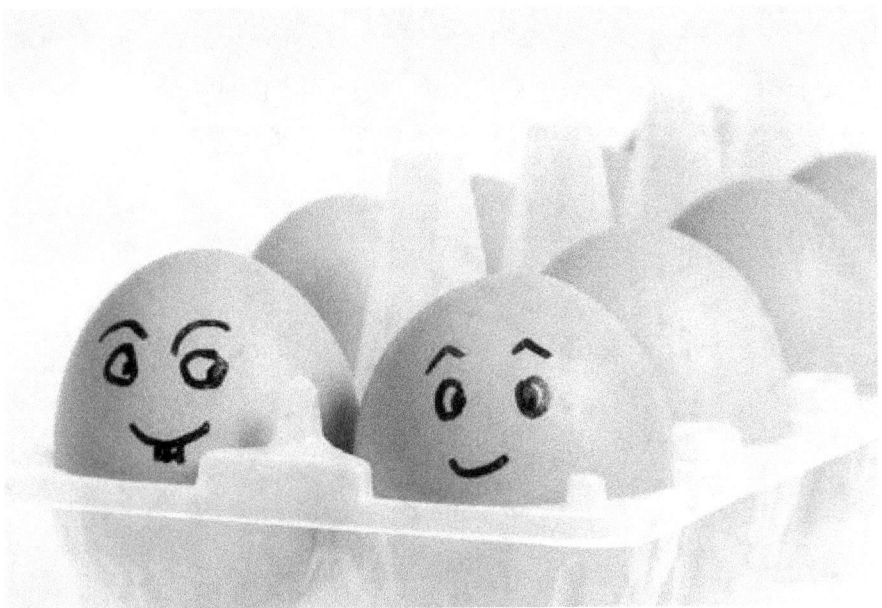

Whenever possible, buy eggs that have been kept under refrigeration. Put them in the refrigerator as soon as possible after you have purchased them. Leave them in the carton with the large end up in a covered container.

Tips on Cooking Eggs

If the eggs are cooked in water, cook under boiling point. If they are baked or fried use low temperatures, high heat will make them tough and unappetizing stop.

Poached Eggs

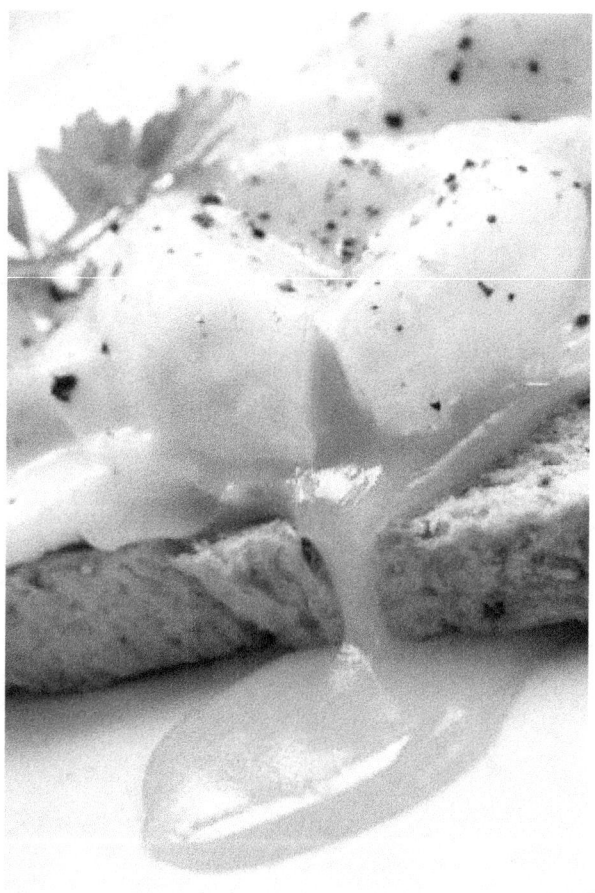

F

ill a shallow pan or frying pan, three quarters full of boiling salted water. Bring the water back to a boil. Break the egg into a saucer, then slip it gently into the water. Repeat with other eggs. A well-drained, attractively poached egg is cooked below the boiling point in salted water.

Reduce heat and simmer, covered, for 3 to 5 minutes or until **the eggs are** set to the desired firmness. Lift the eggs out of the water with a slotted spoon or an egg lifter. Drain well and serve on a warm plate on hot buttered toast.

Eggs can be poached an hour or so before they are to be served and kept warm without changing their texture at all, by placing them in plain lukewarm water.

Fried Eggs

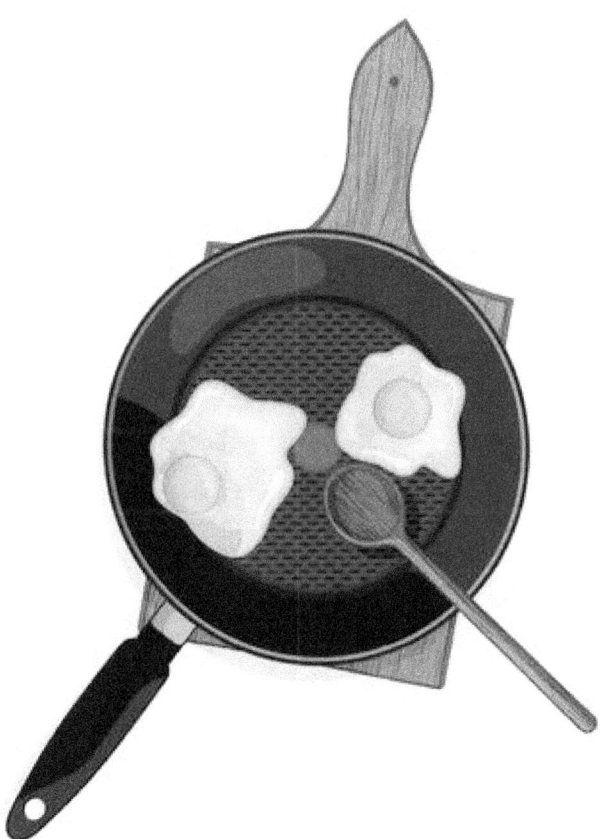

Fried eggs are delicious when they are fried in the fat which is left over after you have already fried bacon. Slide the eggs gently from a saucer into the hot fat.

Turn off the heat to cook the eggs slowly for 3 to 4 minutes. Cover the pan or baste with the fat or turn egg once during cooking, if you are an expert cook to get a pink delicious yolk.

I hate runny yolks, and that is why I do the spooning of hot fat on the egg, – with the heat turned off – before dishing it up on hot buttered toast, with bacon.

Scrambled Eggs

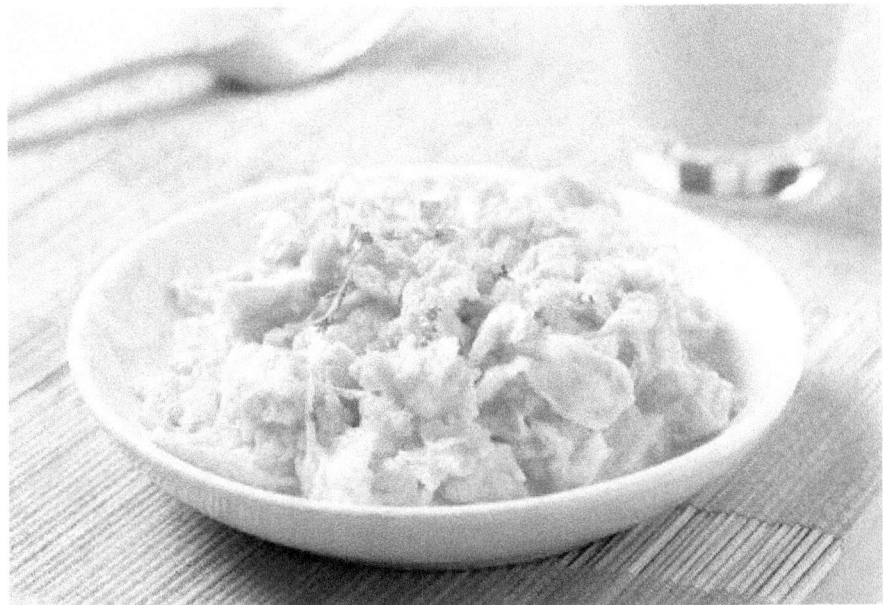

The best fluffy scrambled eggs are cooked over low heat, with plenty of butter. These can be cooked in a skillet or in a double boiler over hot water. You may want to use a double boiler. Not only do they keep hot, but they also keep creamy and moist when the breakfast eaters do not rise at the same time!

To make them really creamy and smooth, stir with a wooden spoon as they cook.

If these scrambled eggs become too rubbery or firm, a little butter or cream or the yolk of another egg can be whipped into them briskly and they will bring back the creaminess.

The addition of some water is going to give you fluffier eggs. Cream is going to give you a richer scrambled eggs mixture.

Scrambled eggs are best, when you add chopped herbs, chopped ham, onions, mushrooms, smoked salmon, and anything else you want to make really delicious and creamy breakfast, healthy dishes. You can add them to the eggs before cooking or right after you pour the eggs into the pan.

If you are going to add cheese while the eggs are cooking, you are going to have streaks of melted cheese in the egg mixture. Either way is delicious.

Traditional French Scrambled Eggs

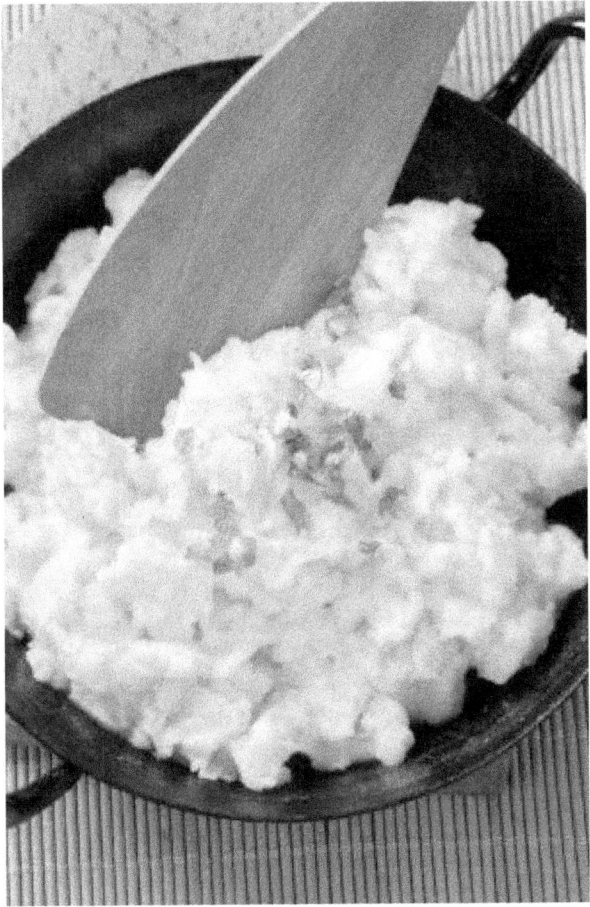

In the frying pan, melt 1 teaspoonful of bacon fat or butter for each egg. Beat the eggs until the whites and the yolks are well mixed. Season with salt and pepper and add 1 teaspoonful of cream or milk, for each egg.

Pour the mixture into the hot fat and cook slowly. Stir gently until the mixture thickens, but is still moist. Serve at once.

As a child I remember watching my great aunt cooking scrambled eggs for breakfast. She used to pour in the egg and the milk mixture in the frying pan and then switch off the heat. After that, she covered the egg pan for just about 25 seconds, – the time it took to butter hot, fresh toast – and then she would put the piping hot egg mixture over the hot buttered toast.

She said the time it took for one to carry your plate to the breakfast table would be enough to cook the scrambled eggs to perfection. Now that was high-quality cookery!

Managing Egg Mixtures

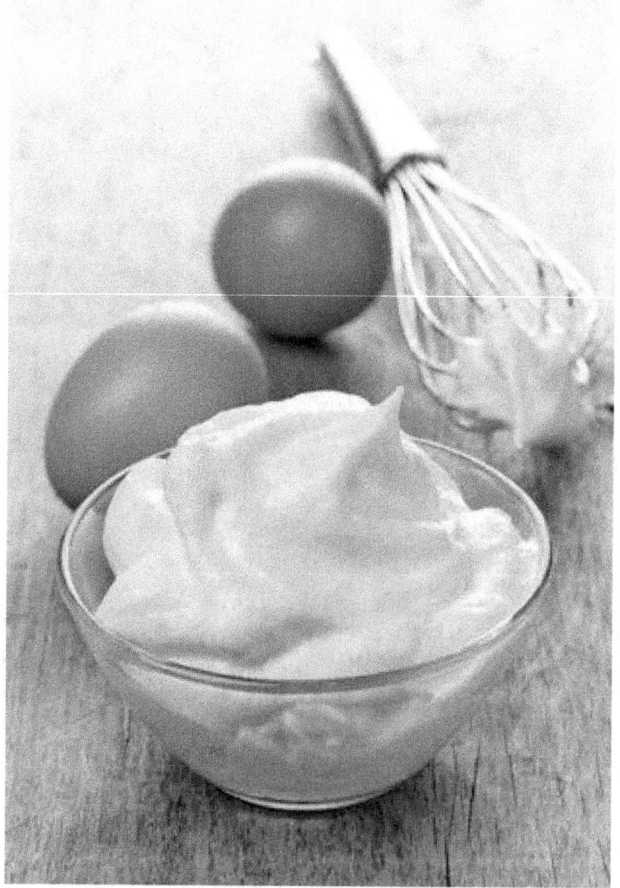

Eggs and egg mixtures should always be cooked over low heat on moderate heat if you want them to be tender. Overcooked eggs are going to be rubbery instead of spongy.

Did you look at any mayonnaise recipe, which asks you for egg whites only? That means just egg whites. Always remove any yolk which gets into the whites when you are separating these eggs. Even a speck of yolk is going to prevent these eggs from beating up to full volume. Only totally white eggs can be beaten up in stiff peaks.

Always put the eggs into the refrigerator as soon as you get them fresh from the store. Eggs lose their quality if they are left for too long in a warm kitchen. Store them broad – side up.

Leftover yolks can keep for two – three days if you covered them with cold water and store them in the refrigerator. Drain and measure 1 1/3 tablespoons for each yolk in recipe.

Remember that there is absolutely no substitute for fresh eggs, and definitely not egg powder. However, egg whites are going to beat up to better volume if they are a bit stale and older.

Eggs cannot be frozen in their shells. You can break all eggs into a jar and freeze them, or you can separate them. For each cup of whole eggs, or yolks, just add 1 teaspoon full of salt. I do not like corn syrup, but one tablespoonful of corn syrup has also been used efficiently as the freezing and preserving agent. Mix thoroughly but do not beat.

Do not add anything to the whites, just put in a container, cover and freeze.

Beating Egg Whites Successfully

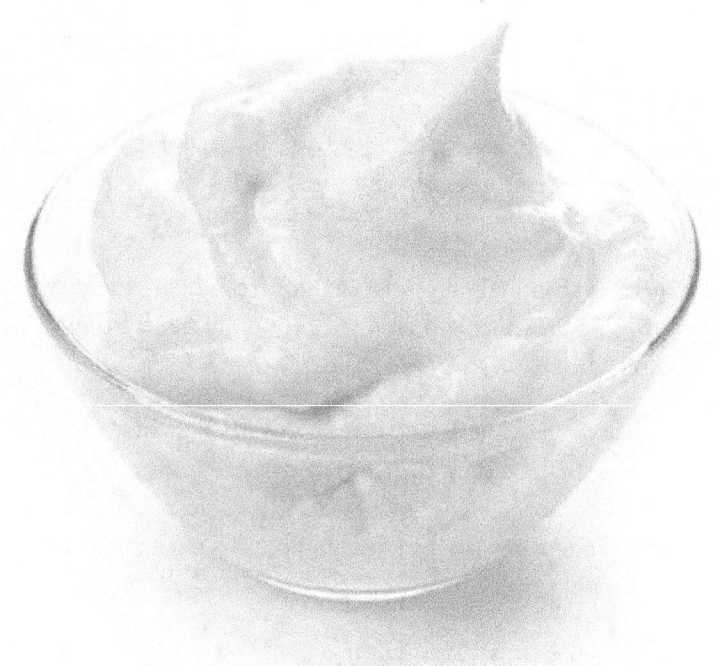

It is easier for you to separate egg whites from the yolks when they are cold, but to beat egg whites to their maximum volume, the beaters, the bowl and the egg whites should have been standing at room temperature for at least half an hour to one hour. Make sure that the beaters as well as the bowl are free from grease.

Do not use plastic bowls, as is very common, because they tend to retain grease.

You may want to add a few grains of salt to the egg whites and beat them to a stiff foam if you are beating by hand. Or you may use the stabilizer which has been used for centuries in the form of ¼ teaspoonful of cream of tartar to six egg whites.

You can also strengthen beaten egg whites by adding 2 tablespoons full of sugar to one egg white, adding 1 tablespoon at a time, sprinkling lightly on the surface and beating constantly. This is done until the mixture stands in peaks and the sugar is dissolved.

Basic Egg Omelette

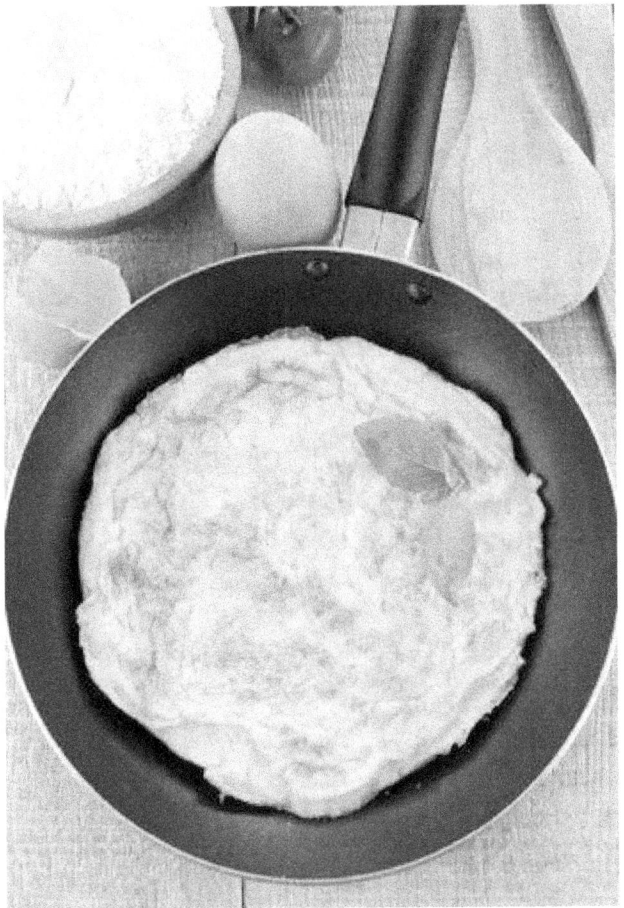

3 eggs, salt and pepper, 6 table spoons milk, and 3 tablespoons butter.

Beat the eggs thoroughly in a bowl. Add salt, pepper, and milk. Then place the butter in the frying pan and melt it. Pour in the mixture. Cook it slowly, lifting the edges of the cooking egg towards the center of the frying pan. Keep tipping the pan. Fold half of the omelette, over the other and serve immediately.

How to Cook Eggs in the Shell

Soft Cooked Eggs

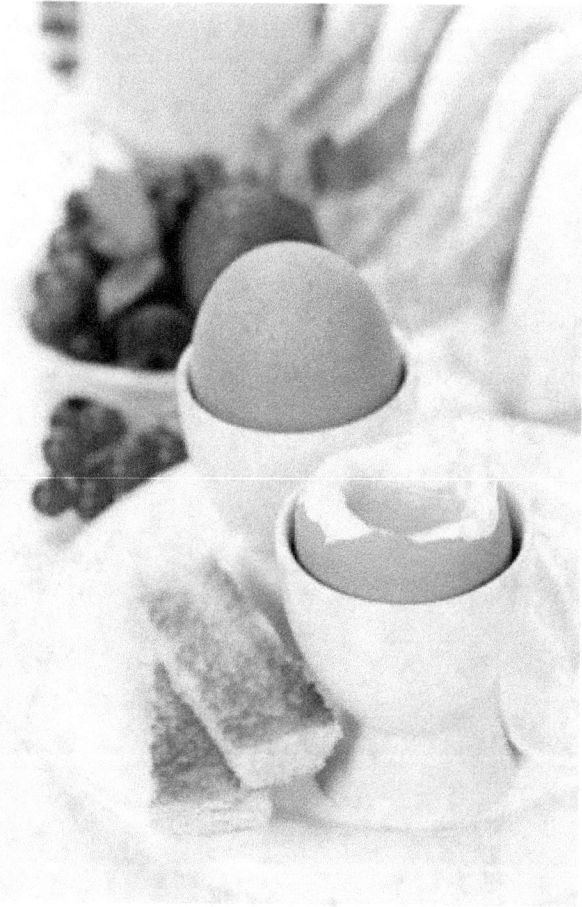

Since ancient times good cooks advocated that eggs in the Shell should not be boiled but they should be cooked to below boiling water temperature for best results. This is done to get tender whites which are firm.

For that you need to place required numbers of eggs in a pan, cover to a depth of 1 in. above the eggs with cold water.

Bring the water to a bubbling boil. Large and active bubbles should be seen rising to the surface. Turn off the heat at once or set the pan off the burner, where the water will keep hot but will not continue to boil.

Cover the pan and let stand for three – 20 minutes depending upon the degree of doneness required.

Three minutes are going to produce a set white and a soft yolk, four minutes produces a slightly set yolk. In fact, one of my friends told me a spiritual way in which her family had been boiling eggs for breakfast down the ages. She had learned this trick from her grandmother. She used to put water on to boil, and then slip the eggs into them. After that, she said the 23rd Psalm and by the time she had finished it, the eggs were done to the best consistency her family enjoyed for breakfast.

I am not a Christian, but what is to prevent me to start the morning with powerful prayers, even unto the 23rd Psalm, especially when I am cooking breakfast for my family? So according to your religious persuasion and denomination, you can say any prayer, depending on the time taken and there you are, a morning prayer said in Thanksgiving and your eggs done perfectly.

You can also cover the eggs with cold water and bring to a boil. There is always the danger that the eggshell is going to crack. So put a little bit of salt in the water or even some vinegar. If the eggshell is already cracked, just put some vinegar in the water and you are not going to have spreading egg.

Remove at once for soft cooked or coddled eggs. For medium cooked eggs, remove the pan from the heat and leave eggs in the water for 3 – 5 more minutes.

Hard cooked Eggs

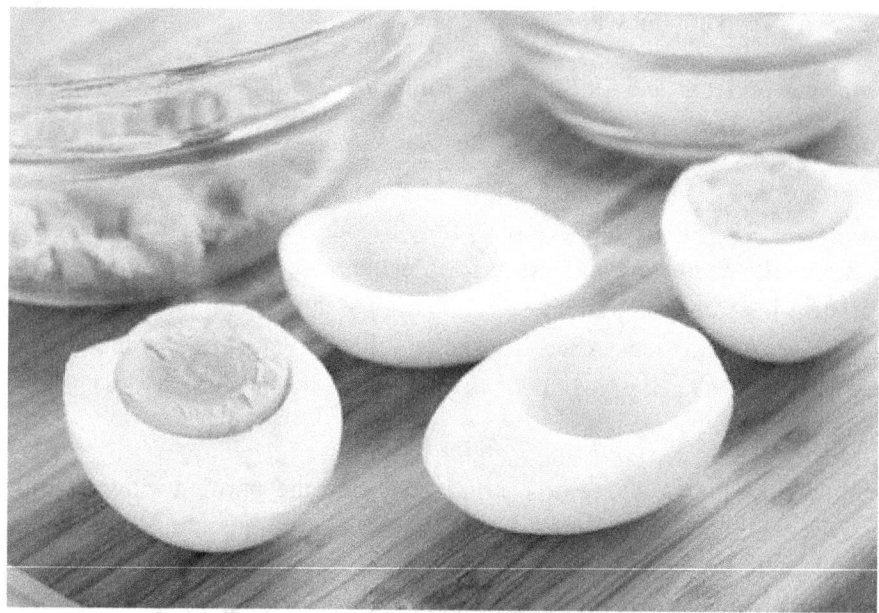

15 minutes should be allowed for hard cooked eggs which have been at room temperature. 20 minutes for refrigerator cold eggs will do perfectly. It is going to take you a little time and experience to look for accurate timing after the water has come to a boil. This is the secret of having eggs in the Shell the way you want it every time.

To stop further cooking of soft eggs when removed from the pan, dip them quickly into cold water, then serve at once, in egg cups.

Hard cooked eggs should be chilled rapidly in cold water to help prevent a dark ring from forming around the egg yolks. I used to wonder whether there was something wrong with the eggs, because I often saw these dark rings in hard-boiled eggs, especially during picnics. It is only now that I learned that you needed to chill them under a running cold water tap, after you took them out of the pan so that there were no dark rings.

This ring was caused by too long cooking or too high a temperature. Prompt cooling will prevent overcooking. It will also help prevent the dark ring, which sometimes appears around the Yolk and help the eggshell come off more easily. You can peel the egg easily by starting to peel it at the large end of the egg.

Here is another easy way in which you can cook a number of eggs at the same time, especially when you want them hard-boiled.

Just put them in a pressure cooker. As pressure cooking is a major part of modern Asian cuisine, this is an excellent way in which we managed to save time while getting a number of items cooked simultaneously in just one large pressure cooker. Place the required number of eggs on a trivet in the bottom of the cooker.

Add half a cup of water. Cover and cook at 5 pounds pressure for eight minutes. Cool the cooker at once under running water. Remove eggs and plunge into cold water.

I normally hard-boil a large number of eggs at the same time, and then place them in my refrigerator, ready at hand for garnishing, chopping up for sandwiches, or just for making a quick egg curry or boiled egg and cheese mixture, whenever necessary. Try it out right now!

Making the Perfect Omelette

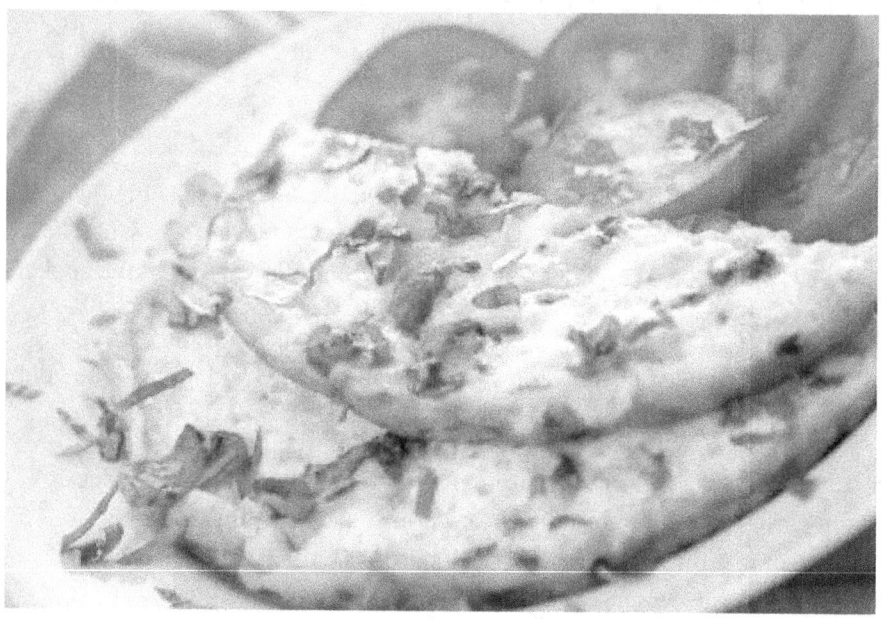

Omelettes are going to be better cooked, if you cook them individually in small skillets – 6 – 8 inches across. That is because the large omelette is unwieldy and difficult to make well. Too much beating of eggs will always make a heavy, watery and poor omelette.

The beating of eggs should be done after the eggs have been broken up well, but that is all unless you want well beaten egg whites for an exceptionally high, and puffy omelette.

You should never use your omelette pan for any other purpose. Do not use any detergent to scrub it. I know of many professional cooks who have seasoned their omelette pans so perfectly, that it will not need to be cleaned, except by wiping out the interior with a paper towel, and adding a little salt to scrub off the stubborn spots.

Never use soap and water to clean these omelette pans, and you are going to have perfect omelettes which are not going to stick to the bottom.

French Omelettes

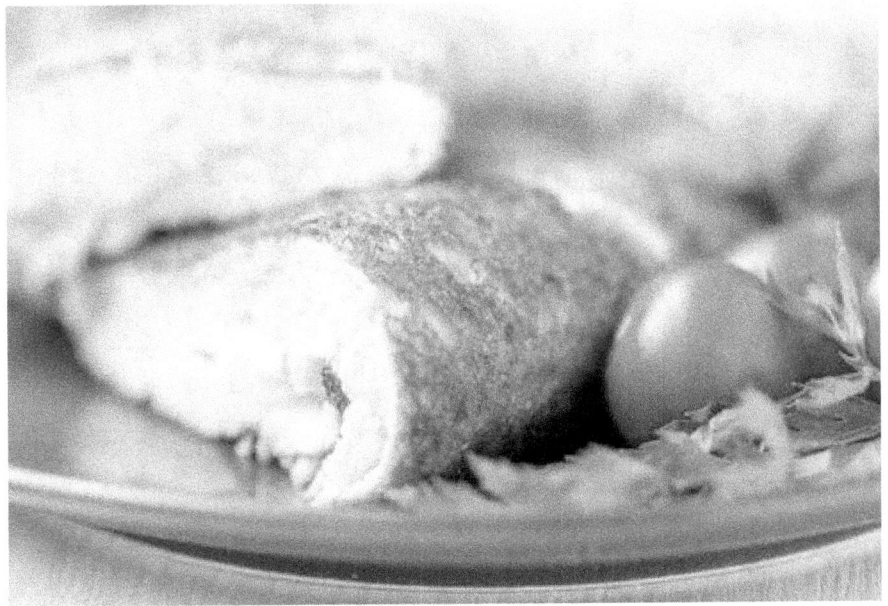

Basic French omelette – bacon fat, 5 eggs, 5 teaspoonful cream or milk, half teaspoonful salt and few grains of pepper.

Melt the fat in the frying pan, beat the eggs, only enough to mixed white and you ask. Add the seasonings and the liquid and then the egg mixture into the frying pan. Reduce heat. As the omelette cooks, prick the bottom and raise the sides to let the liquid portion on the top run underneath until the egg is cooked.

When the bottom of the omelette is lightly browned, fold and turn out on a hot platter. Garnish with parsley. Serve at once to 4 hungry people.

For more hearty and filling French omelets, we use six egg whites, beaten in 6 tbsp. water. In another bowl, we combine the yolks and the salt and pepper, keep beating until the yolks are frothy. Now fold whites in to the yolk mixture. Place the butter in a frying pan and melt it. Let it cook slowly over low heat for one minute until the bottom of the omelette is slightly browned.

Place the frying pan under a grill until the top is slightly brown. Fold it in to half and serve immediately.

Spanish Omelettes

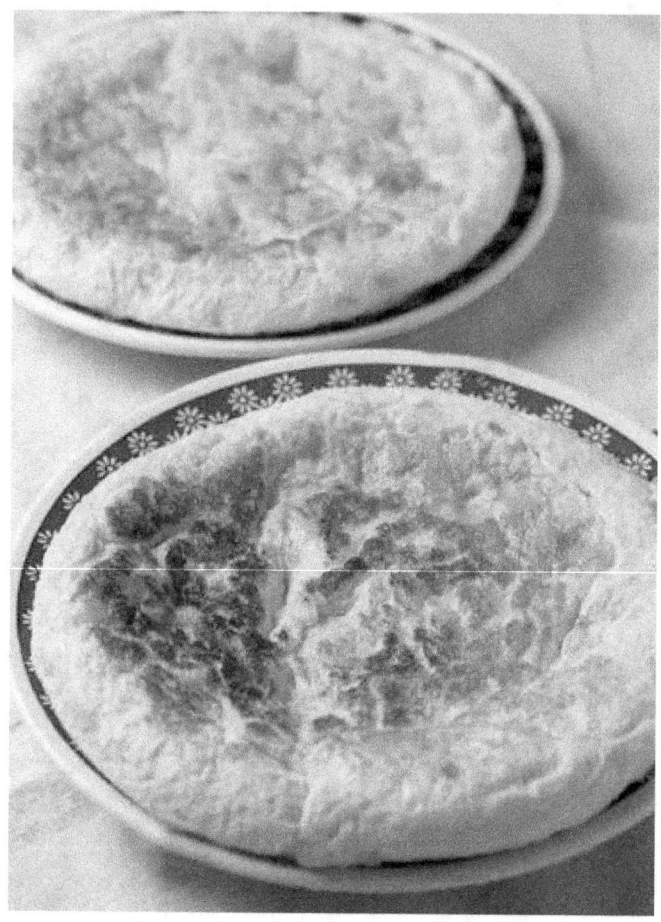

The Spanish omelette is normally given when a hungry person feels like having a hearty meal. That is because it is going to be large, and is going to be stuffed with delicious and nutritious ingredients.

You need five double spoons of oil, three fourths cup chopped onions, half cups chopped green peppers, 3 tomatoes in a paste, salt pepper and chillies to taste, four eggs and half a cup of milk.

In a frying pan cook the onions and the green peppers in the oil. Then add the tomato paste, water, salt and chillies. Cover and bring to a boil. Lower the heat and uncover.

Cook this mixture for eight or 10 minutes. In the bowl, combine the eggs, milk salt and pepper. In another frying pan, heat some more oil, add the egg mixture and cook it. Lift up the omelette as it sets. Keep tilting the edges until the egg is cooked. Serve it with sauce.

So what is the correct spelling of omelette, you may ask? Well, you can either spell it omelette or omelet, or as they do in the Indian subcontinent as Laamlet. Anybody who thought up that pronunciation for an egg beaten flat had a good sense of humor, because in the vernacular, it means "beaten down to the ground, completely flat. "That was definitely the end result of something being whipped into shape and then spread over a flat surface!

Making Perfect Custards

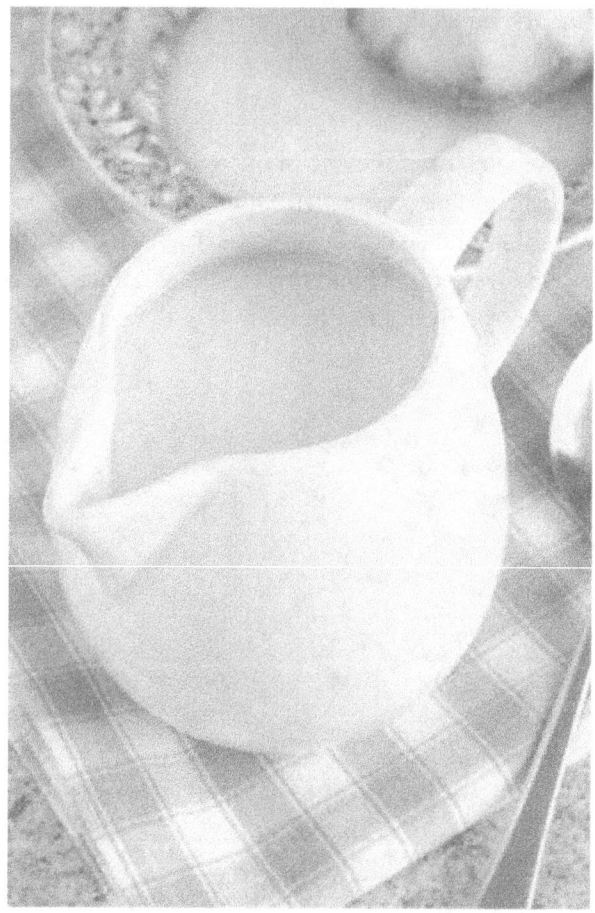

When making a custard, you need to pour hot milk, very gradually on the egg and sugar mixture, stirring all the time. This custard must be cooked over simmering water, or over the lowest heat of your electric unit or gas burner.

Stirring constantly is necessary during the cooking, and keep a watch for signs of thickening.

The time required is going to vary from 6 – 8 minutes for 2 cups of soft custard, and one usually uses a metal spoon for stirring. Just as the custard begins to thicken, the liquid is going to exert a slight drag, and to show faint traces of a sort of a wake while you stir, so you know that the custard has begun to thicken.

The spoon is now going to be coated with the custard.

If custard is baked, the dish must be set in a pan of water and the oven heat has to be low enough so that the water does not boil. The best oven heat is 325° – 350° Fahrenheit and the baking should be done for 25 – 30 minutes or until the custard is set.

Run a sharp knife laid into the custard and see if it comes out clean. That means the custard is baked. Even if the custard is a mite wobbly, do not worry, because it is going to set the moment it cools down.

Making Perfect Soufflés

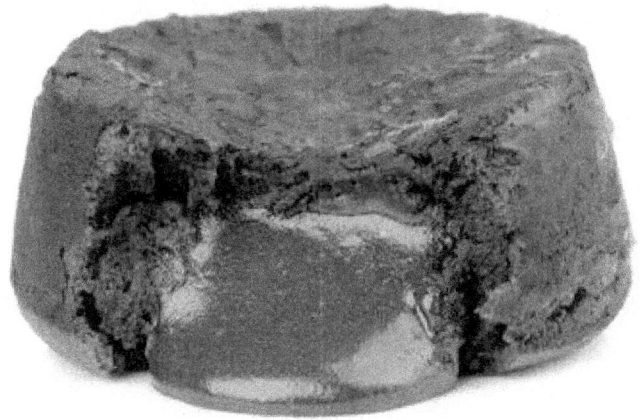

A soufflé has to be handled very carefully and quickly to be good. I remember enjoying a French cartoon[1] of a couple of friends trying to entice one of their melancholy and perpetually depressed friends with a mouthwatering soufflé.

---

[1] Gaston Lagaffe (Gaston the Goof Up) and his cousin Bertrand Labévue (Bertrand the Blunder) the melancholic. There does not seem to be any English translation of this comic.

The words they used were – a perfectly made soufflé has a *je ne sais quoi de la piquante* – and I agree with this sentiment.

Now the soufflé came out of the oven, made to perfection, and the melancholy friend's eyes lit up, only to see the soufflé go down flat with a mumble and a hissssssss. Back went the friend to his state of even darker melancholia and the cook also agreed that he felt a bit flat, himself – no wonder, I would also feel totally *rataplanplan*!

So do not let that happen to you. By using these tips, you can get the perfect soufflés each time, every time.

The yolks must be beaten very light and fluffy and the whites have to be beaten stiff, but not past the point when they begin to lose their sheen and become dry.

Soufflés are usually made with a thick sauce foundation, which may be cooled before being blended with beaten egg yolks. Or you may first try mixing the teaspoonful of water with the beaten yolks, and then a small portion of the hot sauce is mixed with the yolks. When well combined, this can be returned and blended with the hot mixture.

Combining the whites by folding them in is particularly important, and is done by cutting and turning the mixture over and over, very lightly.

Stirring mashes the air out of the whites and the delicacy of the soufflé vanishes.

As soon as the whites are in, the dish must going to the one immediately – every minute of delay is going to give the eggs a chance to go flat.

And finally, everybody must be ready to eat this soufflé the minute it is done!

Egg Cheese Soufflé

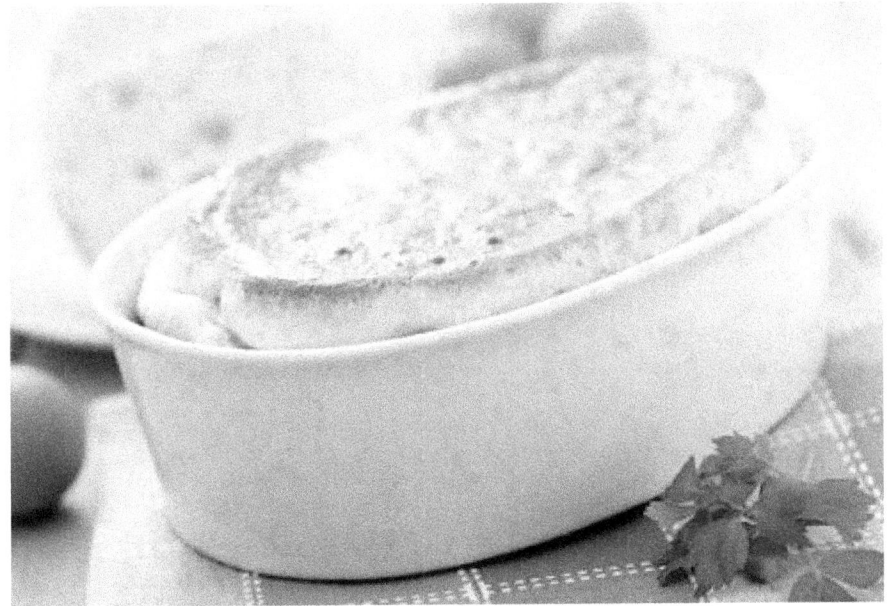

This is a popular Swiss dish, made with 3 tablespoons full of butter, three tablespoonful of flour, 1 cup milk warm, ¼ teaspoon salt, 1/8 teaspoon nutmeg, one Swiss cheese, freshly grated, three egg yolks, three egg whites, 1 teaspoon corn flour.

Melt the butter in the saucepan over a low flame. Blend in the flour. Then add warm milk gradually, stirring constantly, all the while and cook until the mixture is smooth and thickened.

Add salt and nutmeg and stir in the grated cheese. Mix well, remove from heat. Do not allow to boil.

Beat egg yolks until they are thick and lemon colored. Add the cheese mixture, together with the cornflower, stirring, until very smooth. Beat the egg whites until they are stiff and fold in.

Butter a deep baking dish, dust with flour, then filled with cheese mixture. Bake at 350°F for 35 minutes. Serve immediately.

Cheese

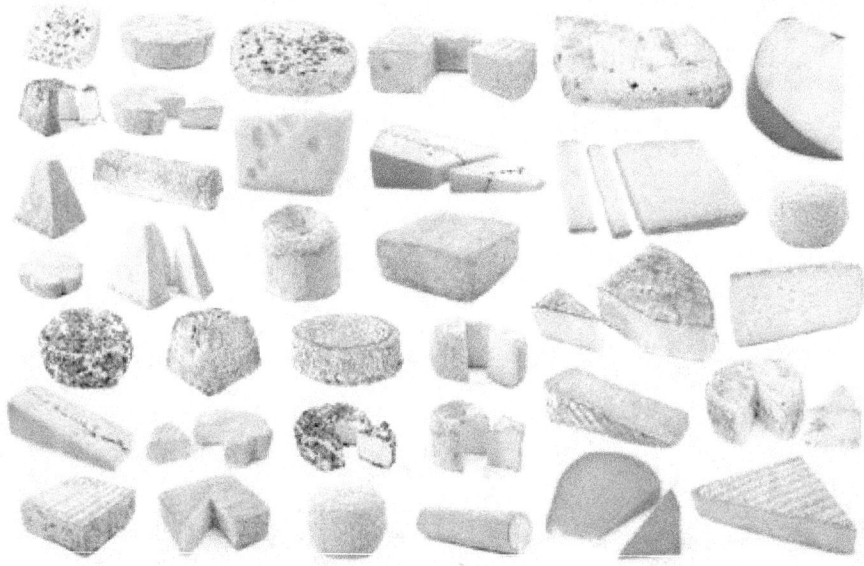

Cheese is a nearly perfect food, like the milk, it is made from. So is it a wonder, that cheese was a regular part of human diet all over the world, since ancient times. It was used in cooking, as well as eaten as it was, sliced, accompanied with bread. In fact, bread and cheese is the staple diet of a number of teenagers, who could not be bothered to prepare breakfast or lunch or dinner for themselves!

In a pound of cheddar cheese, you are going to get the equivalent of milk fat contained in 4 quarts of pure milk.

Cheese is also one of the most versatile of foods, not only fitting in the main course of breakfast and every course of luncheon, or dinner, but it fits every budget. The best thing about cheese is that it is an excellent item for freezing.

There are many excellent varieties of cheese available in the market today. Some of the most popular of the cheeses available to you in the stores are Parmesan, Swiss cheese, Blue,Gouda and pizza – mozzarella cheese from which to choose.

Cheddar cheese is definitely the most popular of available cheeses, globally, and may be purchased as medium cheddar, mild cheddar, or even old cheddar. The flavor of this cheese is going to vary with the length of time the cheese has been aged. It is delicious and sandwiches, on biscuits, or on a cheese and fruit tray. You can also hire date in sauces and casserole dishes. Half a pound of cheese when grated makes 2 cups

Cheddar cheese is made into many varieties of packaged and processed cheese usually sold under brand names. This processed cheese is smooth textured and maybe grated, sliced or used for spreading. I normally do not advocate eating processed foods, especially when they have chemical preservatives in them. So if you can find a place where somebody makes cheddar cheese at home, or any sort of cheese at home, buy it straight from him. At least he is not going to be putting chemicals in it.

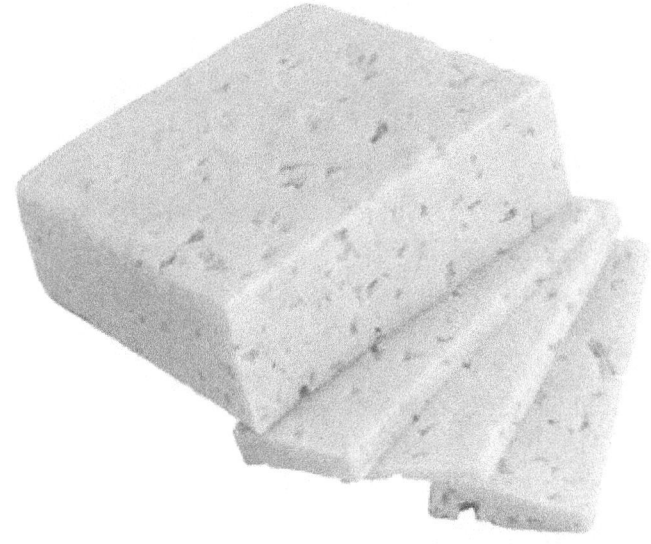

Other hard or semihard cheeses may be used in the same way as cheddar. These include brick cheese, Swiss cheese, and Gouda.

Cottage and Cream Cheese

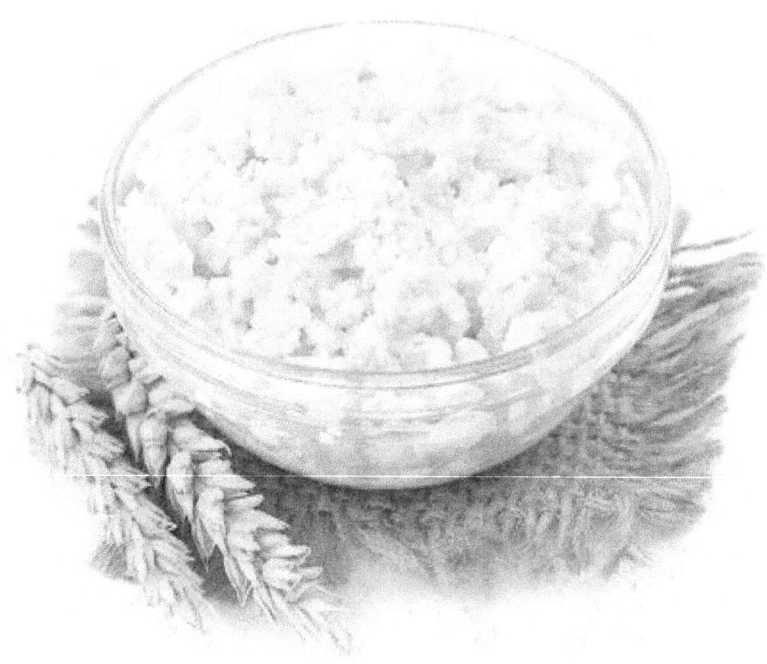

These are the best-known varieties of soft cheese. These cheeses are not aged and are perishable. They may be used for sandwiches, salads, cheesecakes and cheese dips. You may purchase them plain or with a variety of flavorings and seasonings.

In the East, freshly made cottage cheese is made by professional pastry cooks, to be turned into sweetmeats. It is also made into chunks of 1 pound, which you buy, and take home to add to meat and vegetable dishes.

It is easy to make cottage cheese at home.

https://www.youtube.com/watch?v=at8fSKkRKV4

Noreen has some extremely good videos on her YouTube site, – Noreen's kitchen – where you can also learn butter and yogurt. These are also extremely healthy health foods.

You can also try this traditional way of making cottage cheese. For this you need two quarts of sour milk and some cream and salt.

Heat the milk over hot water until it is quite hot –approximately 120°F. The mixture should appear to curdle and thicken.

Remove from heat, leave to stand in a warm place for about half an hour for the curds to collect. Turn into a cheesecloth lined strainer to let the whey drain off thoroughly.

If the milk was very sour, you can pour a quart of warm water over this mass. Repeat again with cold water is necessary – this is when the whey flow is halted – tie in cheesecloth and leave to drain overnight.

When dry, crumble the cheese curds finely and add salt. When serving, add cream and mix thoroughly. This is going to make approximately 2 cups.

You can freshen cottage cheese with 2 cups of sweet milk, and 1 cup of cottage cheese.

Heat the milk until it is hot to the touch – 115°F. Remove from the stove, add the cheese to the milk and stir. Leave undisturbed until cool, then drain in your cheesecloth bag.

Storing Cheeses

Cheese can be frozen and stored in the freezer for a long time. After removal from the freezer, allow it to thaw slowly in the refrigerator, and later reach room temperature before you use it.

I would suggest freezing quantities likely to be used at one time. If you have sliced cheese for sandwiches, before freezing, put two thicknesses of wax paper or freezer wrap between the slices so that they can separate easily.

If you intend to store cottage cheese for any length of time in your freezer, use the un-creamed cottage cheese type.

Dry cheese tip – if your cheese has become too dry, just soak it in buttermilk and it is going to return to normal.

Always remember to keep cheese in an airtight glass jar in the refrigerator and is going to remain fresh for a long long time.

Cheese is not widely used for cooking in Spain, where cheeses are not left to mature, but Spanish egg omelettes are famous as are several versions of an egg, pork and ham baked mixture.

How to Cook Cheese

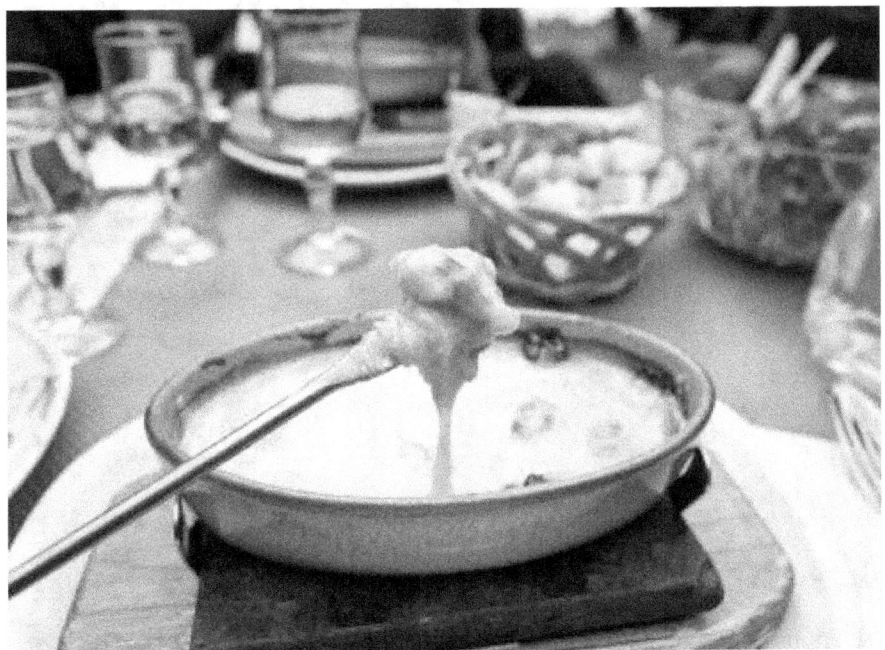

Always cook any food containing cheese at a low temperature, if it has to be cooked for any length of time. Higher temperatures may be used if the cooking time is very short. Over cooking is going to give cheese a bad texture and may be hard to digest.

When you cut cheese, shared or grated and mix it with other foods, there is less danger of overcooking it.

Cheddar which has been well ripened is going to blend more readily than that which is under ripened, and any cheese that has a high fat content is going to melt better than others.

If cheese is going to be served on its own, remove it from the refrigerator and hour or more before it is to be served, so that its full goodness can be released.

Casseroles, which contain eggs, cheese and milk should be poached in a moderately slow oven. [325 – 350°F] . For poaching them in the oven, set the baking dish or the casserole in another pan and surround with hot water.

Here is my favorite cheese spread recipe.

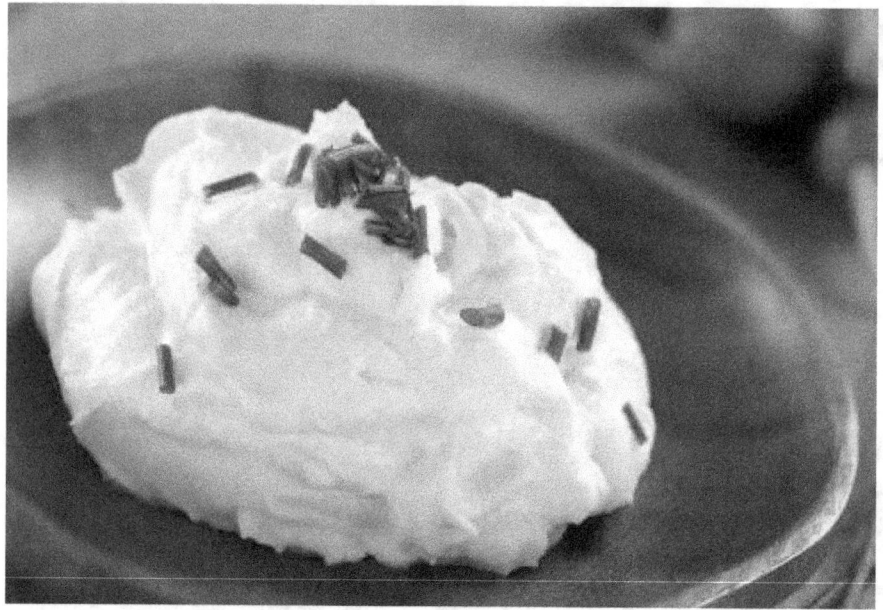

You can make this with leftover cheese, grated and be used instead of butter. Spread it on bread, biscuits, or cakes, or any other available surface.

Half cup cheese, grated, ¼ cup butter, one egg, beaten, 1/3 cup milk, 1/8 teaspoon cayenne, ¼ teaspoon dried mustard, salt to taste.

Combine the cheese and the butter in the top of a double boiler. Melt over hot water and blend. Add the egg, milk, canned pepper, mustard and cook, stirring until thickened and creamy.

Add salt to taste. Pour into a small jar stop. Cool and refrigerate. This is going to keep for a week.

Swiss Toast with Scrambled Eggs

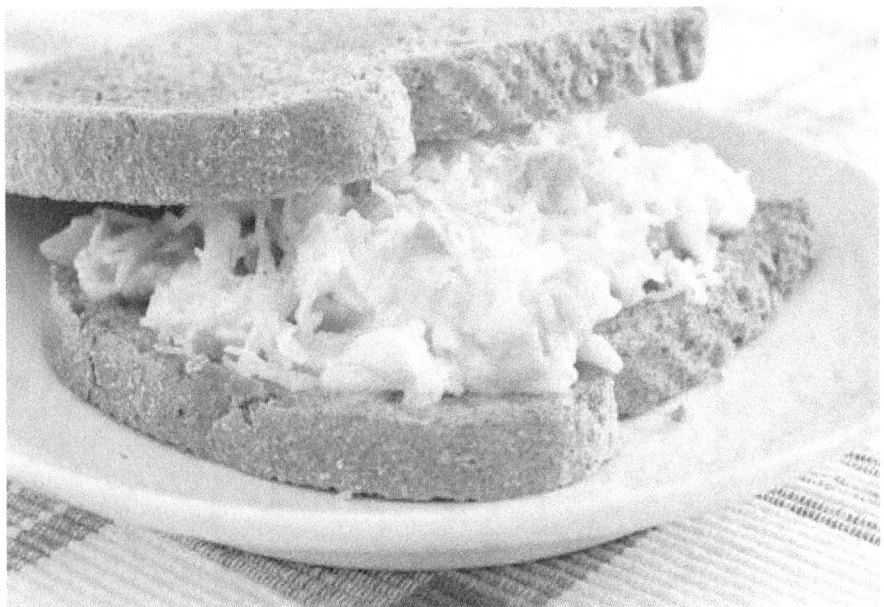

You can also chop up the ham.

Perfect for a breakfast dish. **4 slices bread, butter, four slices cooked ham, four slices Swiss cheese and scrambled eggs.**

Prepare scrambled eggs as per the recipe given above. Toast the bread and spread with the butter. Place slice of ham on each slice of toast. Top each with a slice of cheese.

Brown in the oven at 425°F and serve with scrambled eggs.

Conclusion

This book has given you an introduction to egg and cheese dishes, and how you can use these two highly nutritive foods in delicious combinations, in either dishes you have created yourself or from recipes you have found in this book.

Remember that you are responsible for the ultimate good health of your family, so look for healthy nutritive cheese and eggs and feed them with this good combination often.

Live long And Prosper!

Authors Bio

Dueep Jyot Singh is a Management and IT Professional who managed to gather Postgraduate qualifications in Management and English and Degrees in Science, French and Education while pursuing different enjoyable career options like being an hospital administrator, IT,SEO and HRD Database Manager/ trainer, movie , radio and TV scriptwriter, theatre artiste and public speaker, lecturer in French, Marketing and Advertising, ex-Editor of Hearts On Fire (now known as Solstice) Books Missouri USA, advice columnist and cartoonist, publisher and Aviation School trainer, ex- moderator on Medico.in, banker, student councilor ,travelogue writer … among other things!

One fine morning, she decided that she had enough of killing herself by Degrees and went back to her first love -- writing. It's more enjoyable! She already has 48 published academic and 14 fiction- in- different- genre books under her belt.

When she is not designing websites or making Graphic design illustrations for clients , she is browsing through old bookshops hunting for treasures, of which she has an enviable collection – including R.L. Stevenson, O.Henry, Dornford Yates, Maurice Walsh, De Maupassant, Victor Hugo, Sapper, C.N. Williamson, "Bartimeus" and the crown of her collection- Dickens "The Old Curiosity Shop," and so on… Just call her "Renaissance Woman") - collecting herbal remedies, acting like Universal Helping Hand/Agony Aunt, or escaping to her dear mountains for a bit of exploring, collecting herbs and plants and trekking.

1. Amazon.com
2. Barnes and Noble
3. Itunes
4. Kobo
5. Smashwords
6. Google Play Books

Check out some of the other JD-Biz Publishing books

Gardening Series on Amazon

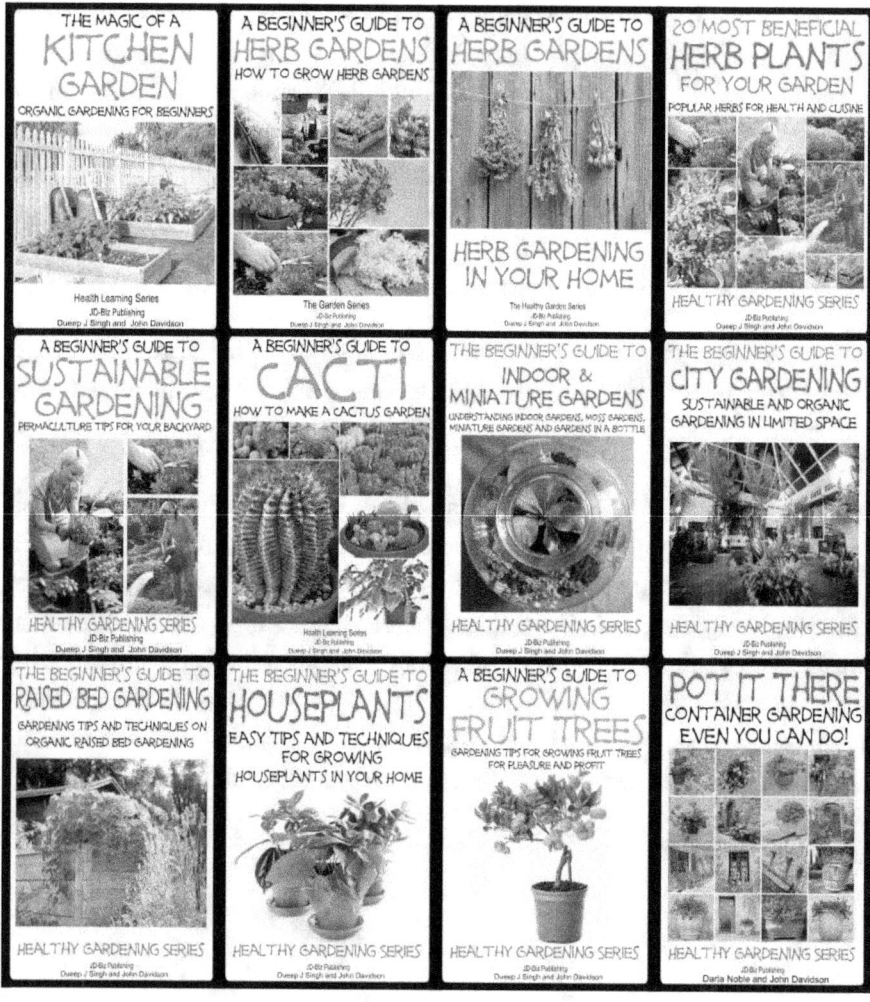

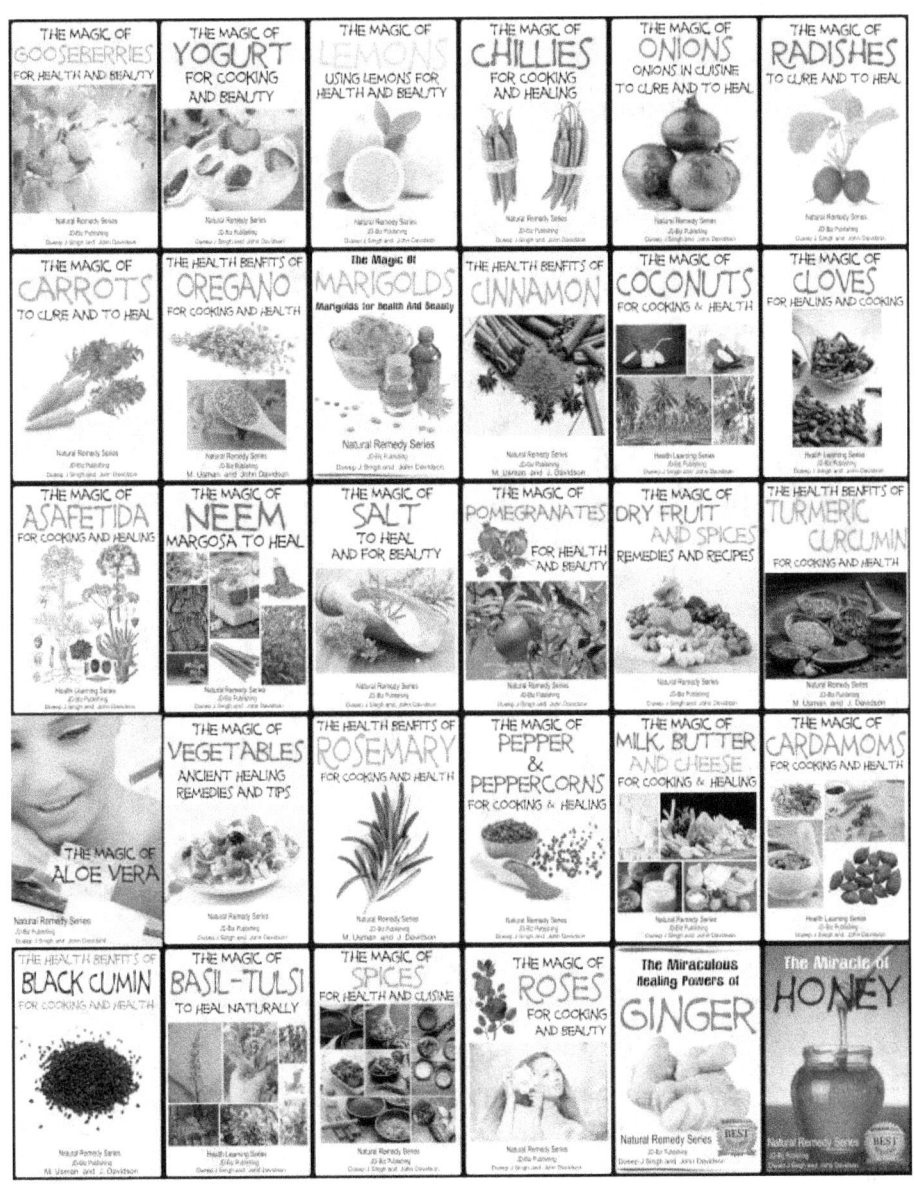

Country Life Books

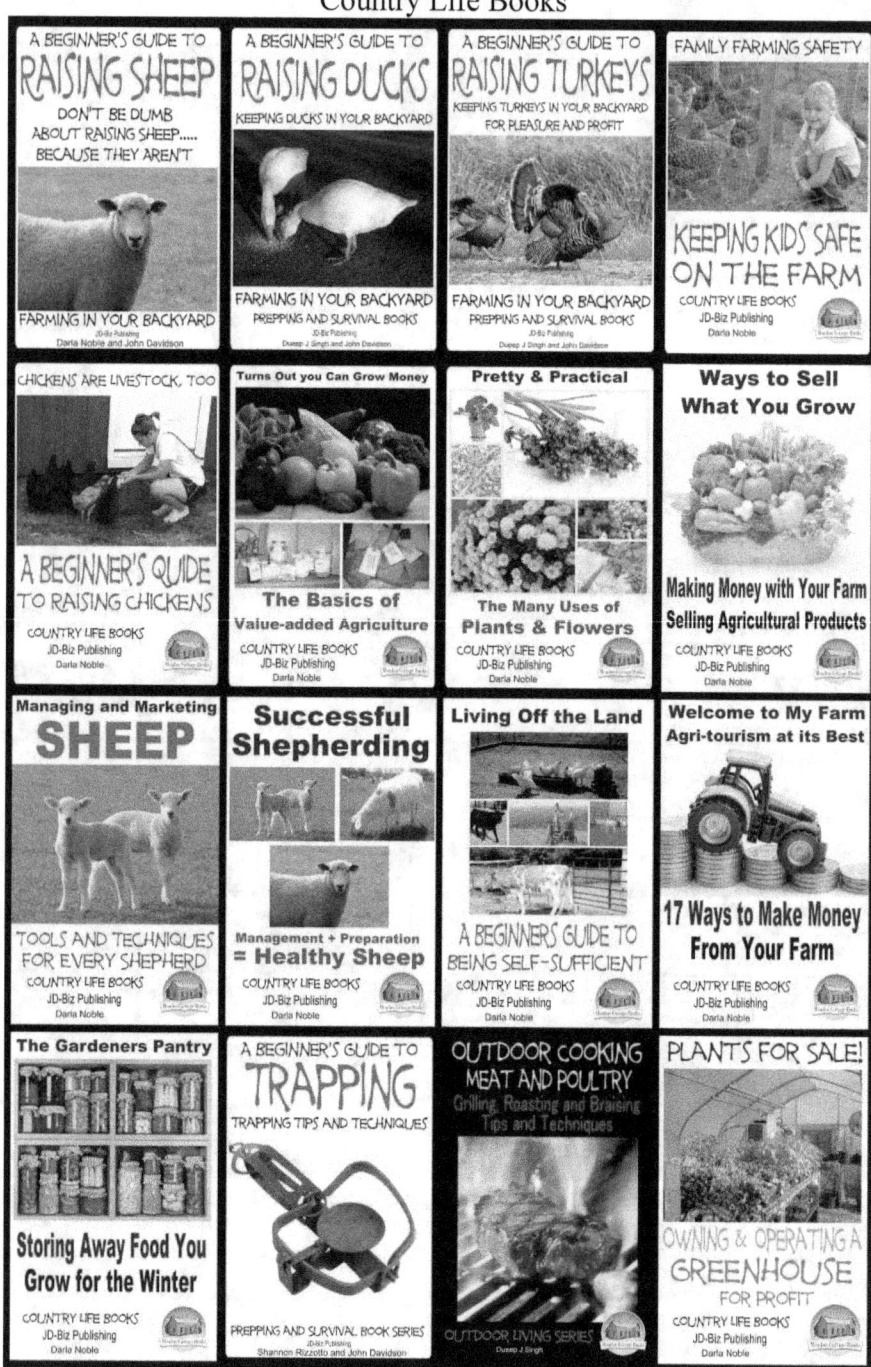

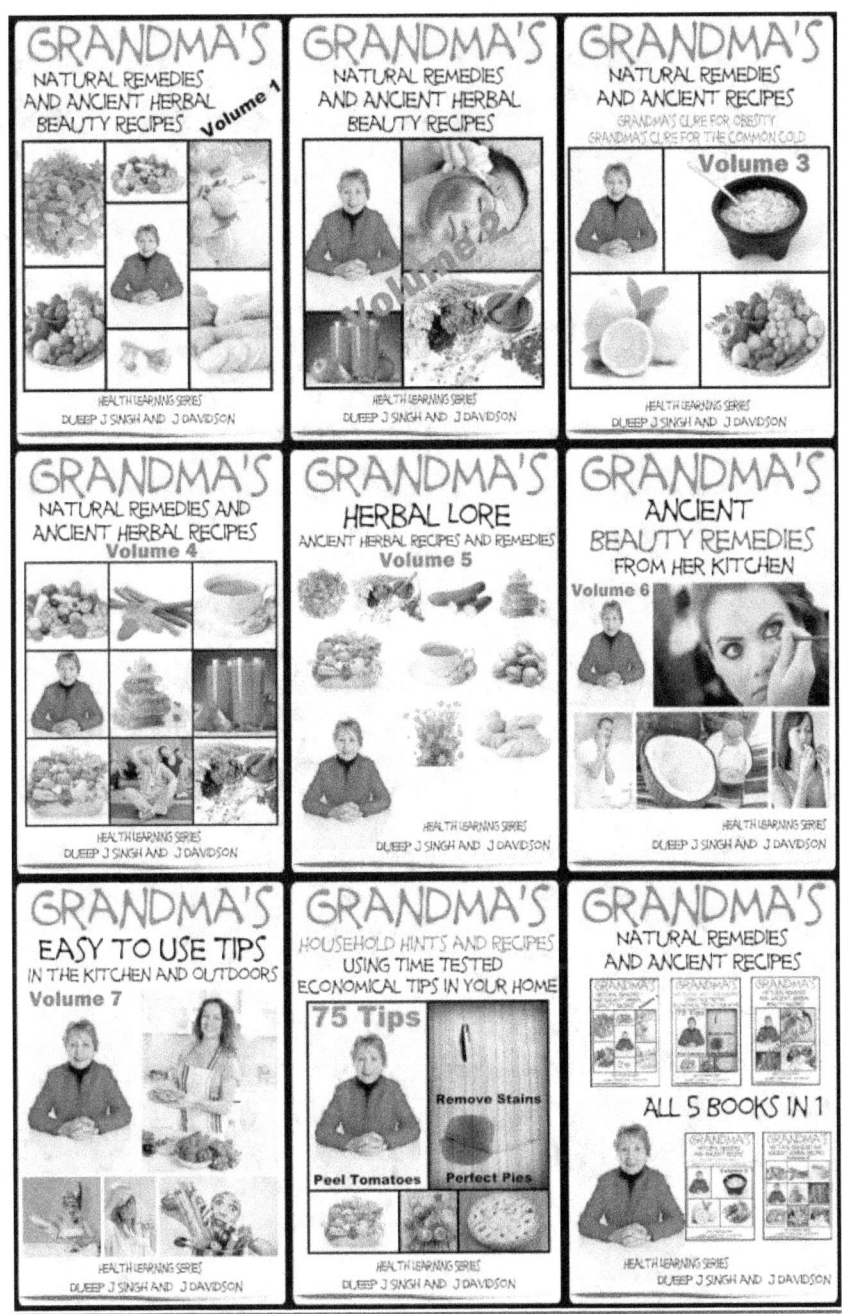

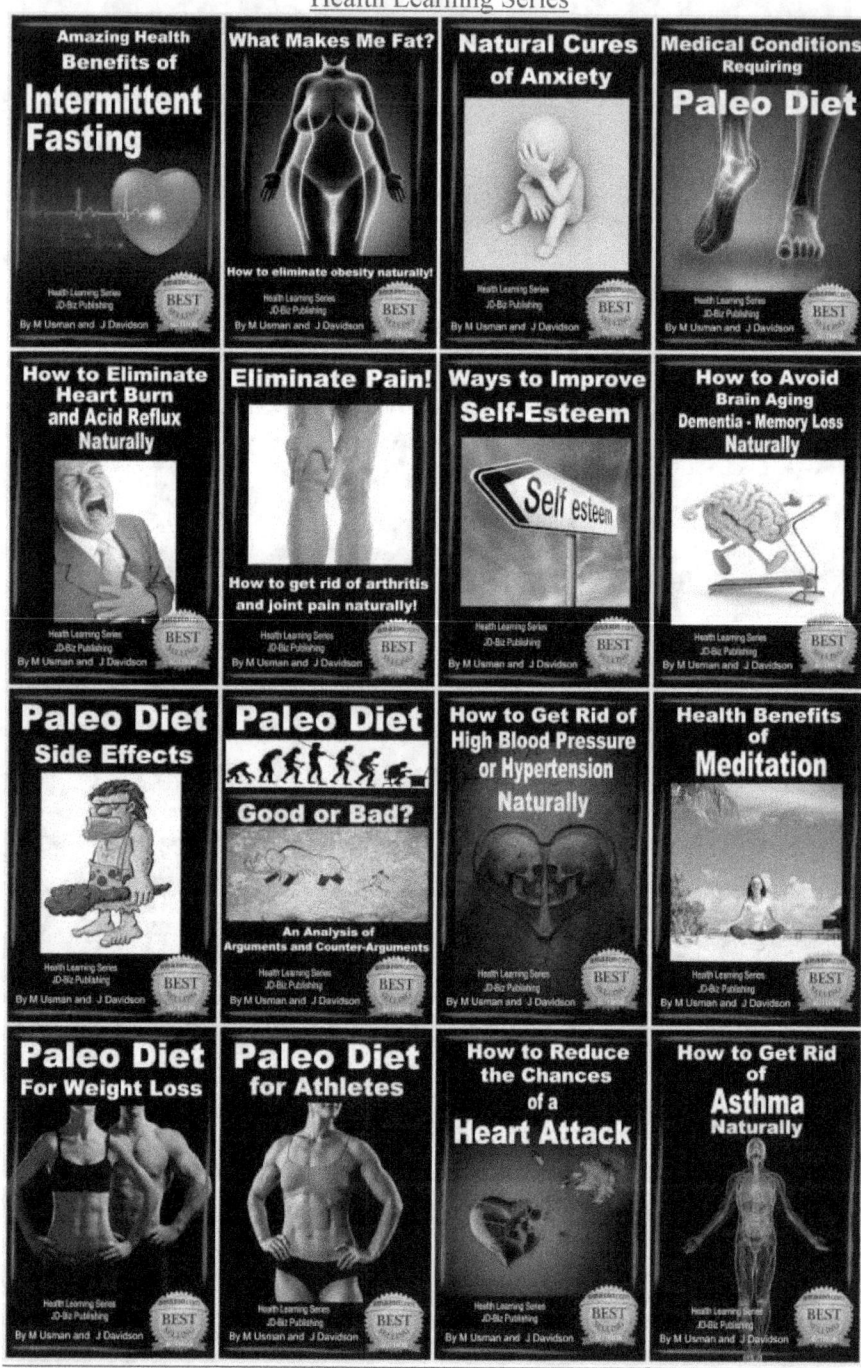

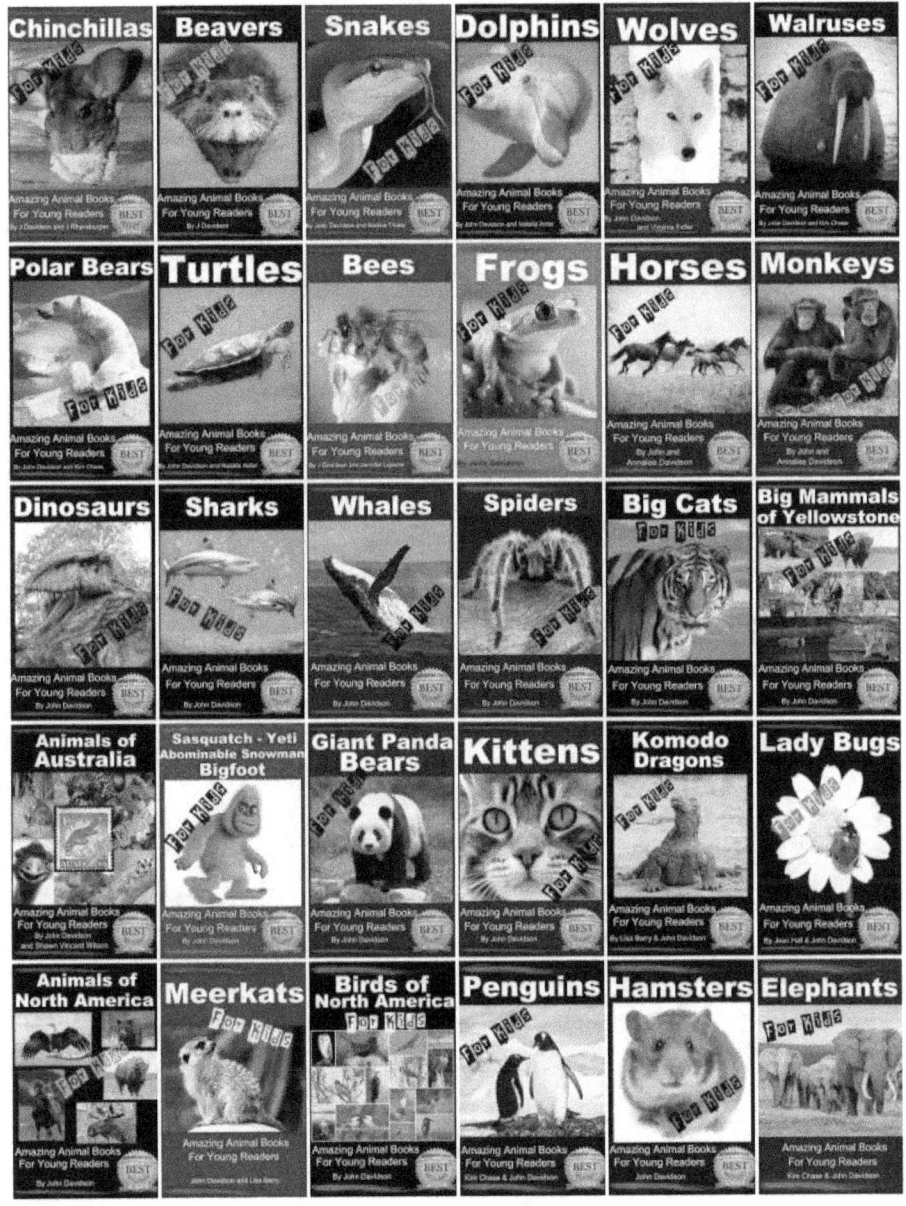

Learn To Draw Series

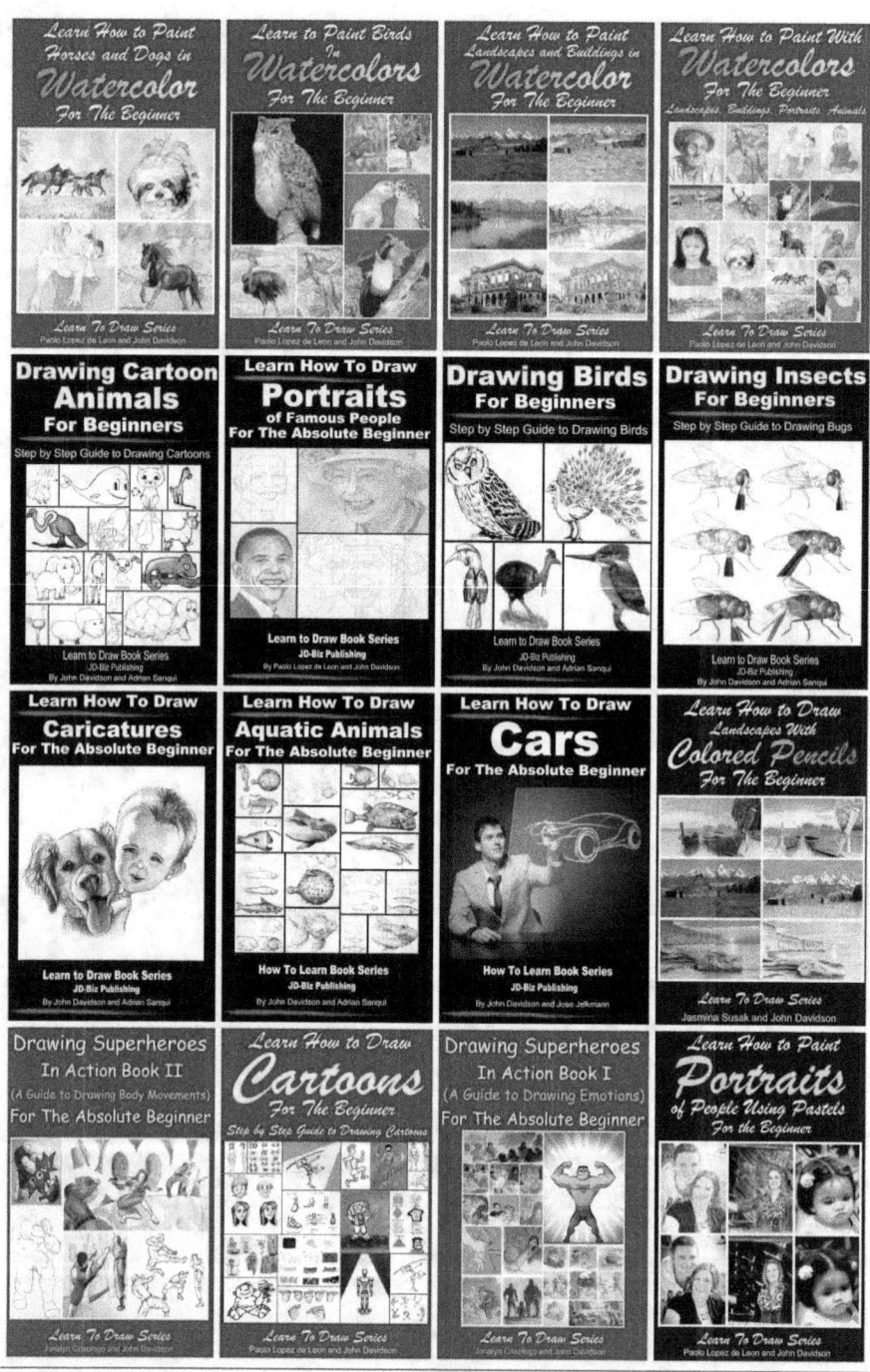

How to Build and Plan Books

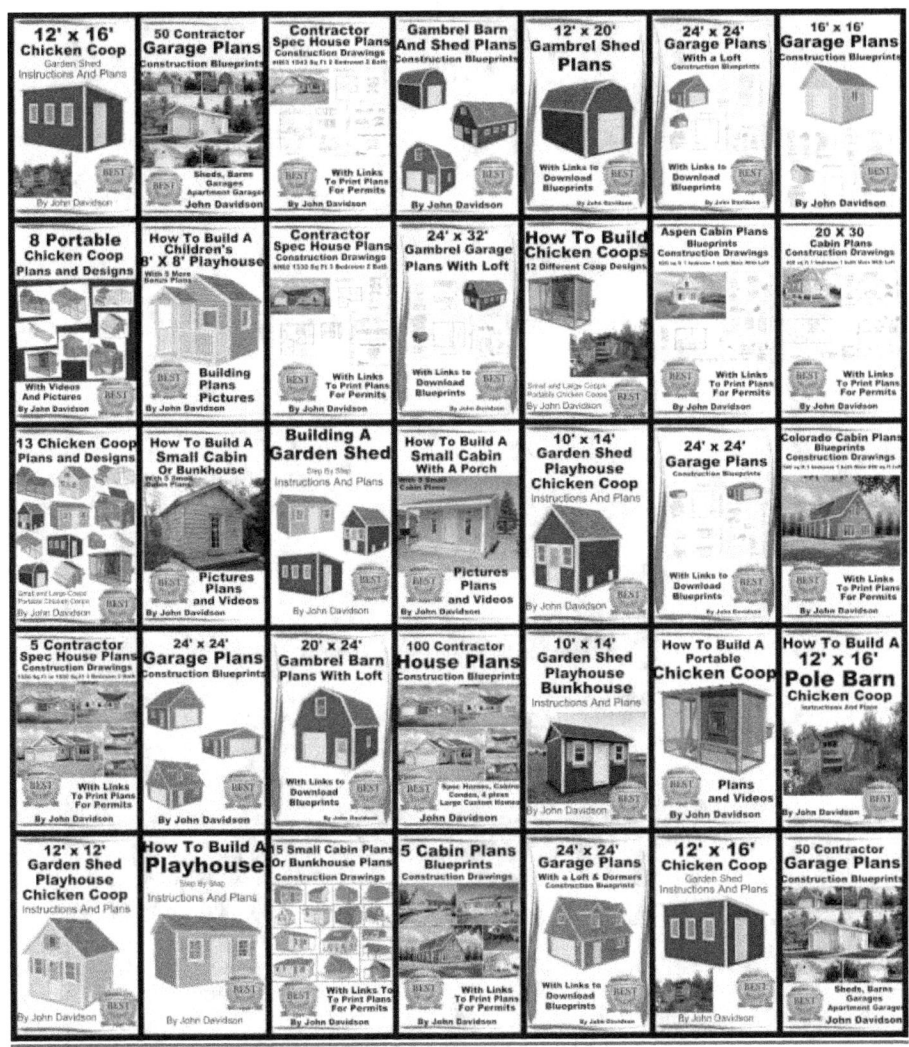

Entrepreneur Book Series

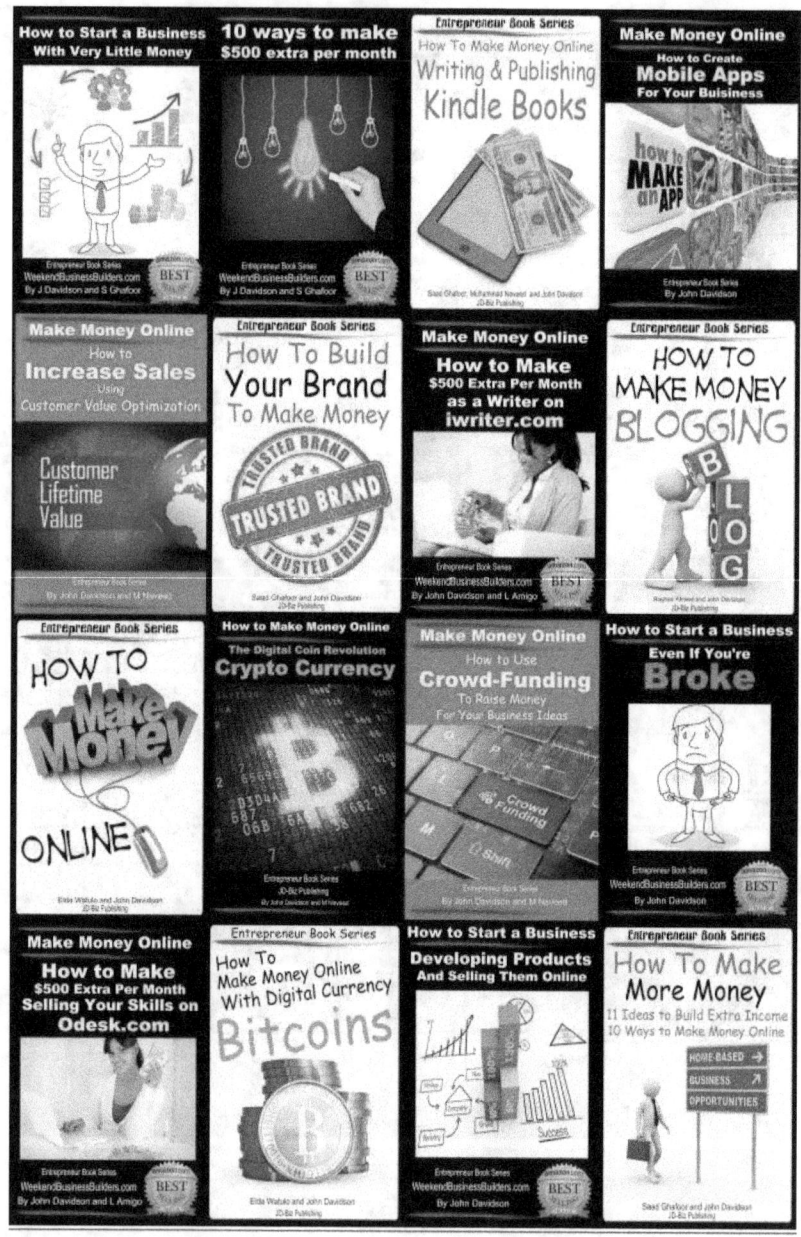

Publisher

JD-BIZ PUBLISHING

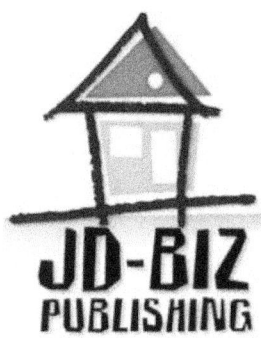

JD-Biz Corp

P O Box 374

Mendon, Utah 84325

http://www.jd-biz.com/

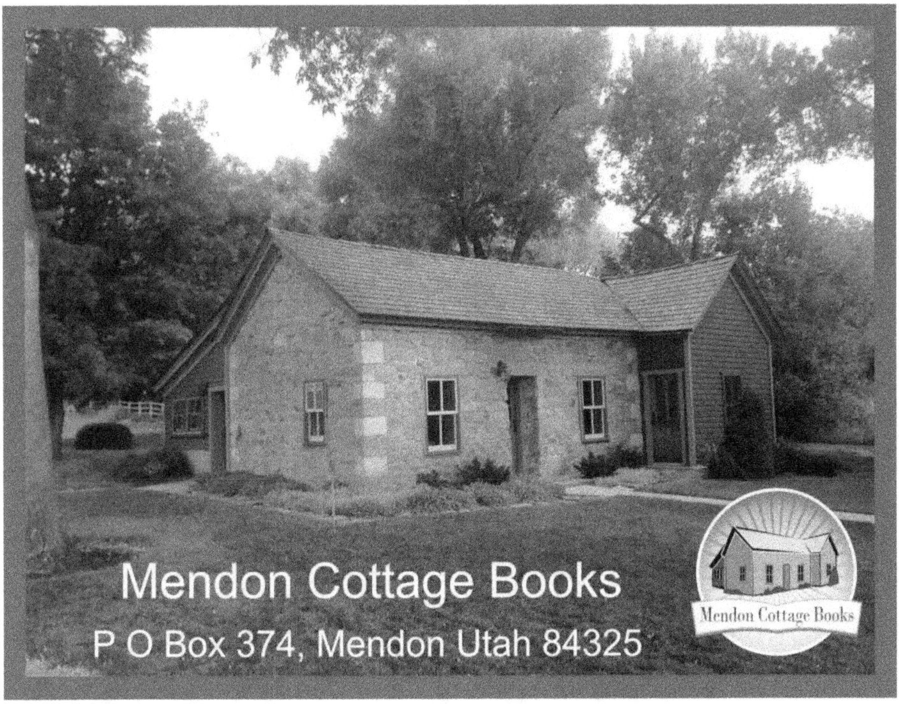

Mendon Cottage Books
P O Box 374, Mendon Utah 84325
Mendon Cottage Books

www.ingramcontent.com/pod-product-compliance
Lightning Source LLC
Chambersburg PA
CBHW071132280526
45787CB00003B/1261